The Mediterranean Diet: A Complete Guide

50 Quick and Easy Low Calorie/High Protein Mediterranean Diet Recipes For Weight Loss

CAC Publishing

ISBN: 978-1-948489-16-4

Matthew A. Bryant

Thank You

The Mediterranean diet is not just a diet — it is a complete lifestyle that will empower you to develop a healthy relationship with food. These easy Mediterranean recipes are fun, quick, and will help you meet your weight loss goals. The Mediterranean diet is also proven[1] to lower the risk of many lifestyle diseases including certain types of cancers, heart disease, Alzheimer's, and Parkinson's disease.

This eBook is dedicated to all those who wish to live well, eat well and take back control of their health.

Make sure to check out my new meal plan titled **The 90 Day Mediterranean Diet Meal Plan for Healthy Weight Loss**. It has 147 DELICIOUS recipes, daily meal plans, and weekly shopping lists for a full 90 days! Every recipe was meticulously crafted with weight loss in mind. It's the most comprehensive meal plan ever assembled so don't miss it! You can get it here: 90 Day Mediterranean Diet Meal Plan

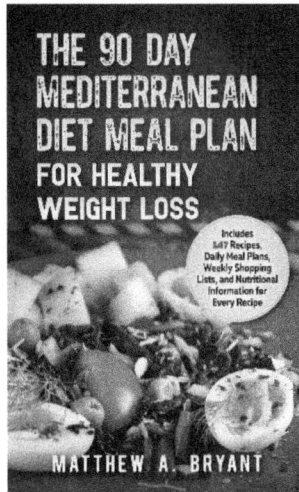

Check out my Facebook group, too! It's a fantastic community of over 6,500 people interested in the Mediterranean Diet. Lots of great information, delicious recipes, and great people! https://www.facebook.com/groups/1023957707694936/

Table of Contents

Introduction

Americans, unfortunately, have a strange relationship with food. Many advertisements and food shows depict standard American fare as plates piled high with bacon, steak, eggs, meats, and a pile of breads, and call it healthy. We are also constantly eating: each and every celebration of ours is about food, be it birthdays, an evening out with friends, and even the formal office lunch meetings. To lose the weight that we have invariably packed on due to these habits, we try to deprive ourselves through dieting. We count calories, we cut carbs, we spend thousands of dollars on weight loss pills — but in the end, we only feel miserable because of the lack of results.

The Mediterranean diet has come to be known as the World's Best Plant-Based Diet[2] to lose weight and prevent a host of chronic diseases, without the need for painfully small portions or eliminating whole food groups. The Mediterranean diet isn't a "diet" at all — at least not in the sense that many Americans understand the word. Rather than a temporary measure to lose weight, it's a series of habits that create lifelong health.

Many people living in Mediterranean countries — namely Spain, Greece, and Italy — have been eating what has become popular today as the Mediterranean diet for generations. The foods in this diet include high amounts of olive oil, legumes, nuts, seeds, vegetables, and whole grains. It also consists of fish and seafood, which are ideally consumed once or twice a week. Eggs, cheese, and yogurt are consumed moderately, about once a week. The intake of red meat and sweets is kept to a minimum. The people of Greece have been eating this way for centuries, and they are known to have lower rates of obesity[3] compared to other countries. The Greeks have a philosophy in life: *everything in moderation*. That is the Mediterranean diet in a nutshell. Today, doctors have uncovered the science behind the long-term health benefits of eating the way Greeks do. Based on extensive research proving the advantages of this diet, many of the world's leading cardiologists[4] are recommending the Mediterranean diet to heart patients.

The Mediterranean diet first arrived in America nearly four decades ago, but it is still highly misunderstood. This book has been written with that widespread misunderstanding in mind. It is written for families with children, single people, for the aging, the elderly with health issues, and for the vast majority of people who can benefit from understanding that the Mediterranean diet is not just about the food we eat, but also about enjoying meals and life with family and friends.

In the first chapter, we will discuss the health benefits of this lifestyle in detail. We will also debunk some myths surrounding this diet and cover the basics of how to start living the Mediterranean way. Then, we will explore 50 delicious recipes for breakfast, lunch, dinner, and snacks.

So let us set sail to healthier hearts, lower BMIs, and a better quality of life!

Chapter 1: Magic of The Mediterranean Diet

What is The Mediterranean Diet?

The Mediterranean diet (or the Med diet, as it is sometimes known) is the name given to the eating habits of people living in the region that surrounds the Mediterranean Sea, including Spain, Italy, and Greece. The inhabitants of these regions are a mixture of Christians, Jews, and Muslims, and each of these religions has added their own distinct flavors to create what is known as the Mediterranean style of eating. For example, Muslims do not eat pork or drink wine; Jews avoid shellfish and pork; Christians drink wine but avoid eating meat on certain days of the week. These dynamic traditions have all shaped the Mediterranean diet into what it is today.

Western interest in the diet started to grow when doctors noticed a trend: people living in and around the Mediterranean region experienced much lower rates of heart disease and obesity than those living in other parts of the world. Scientists discovered higher amounts of Omega-3 essential fatty acids in the diet of people in this region thanks to the high amounts of olive oil in traditional Mediterranean cuisine. Additionally, people in these areas also had a lower intake of solid animal fats like lard. The fats found in nuts and olive oil, which are widely consumed in the diet, were found to be of the monounsaturated or polyunsaturated varieties. Not only did these types of fats fail to raise LDL cholesterol (the bad cholesterol), but they actually increased HDL (the good cholesterol).

The Mediterranean tradition is about more than the ingredients used in its cuisine. Food is looked upon as a representation of life, and all meals are considered to be a social occasion and an opportunity to gather with friends and family. The Mediterranean diet is not just about a set of eating habits, but about developing a healthy relationship with food as part of a fulfilling life.

The Mediterranean Diet Pyramid

The Mediterranean Food Pyramid

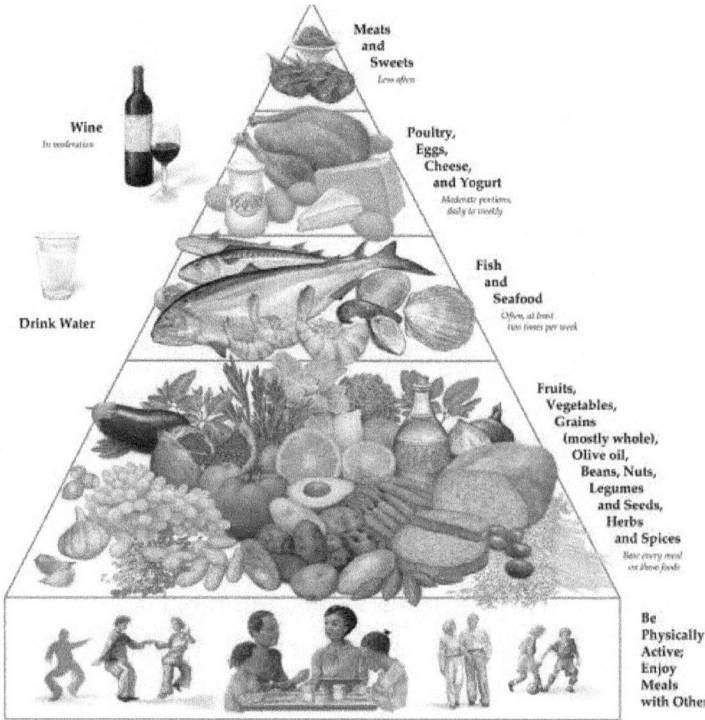

Image source: Old Ways Health Through Heritage

As you can see from the food pyramid, the Med diet is plant-based. The base of the pyramid, which consists of foods that are eaten in the largest relative quantities, is comprised of vegetables, whole grains, nuts, fruits, legumes, beans, seeds, herbs, and spices. Besides these foods, there's another fundamental aspect of the Mediterranean food pyramid: enjoying meals with loved ones and being physically active. Traditionally, the people in the Mediterranean region are known to spend time tending to their gardens, riding bikes, or dancing at social gatherings, with plenty of opportunities to stay active and healthy.

Above the social layer and the basic food groups layer is the tier containing fish and seafood. Seafood is eaten a couple of times a day, with a focus on healthy fish that provide plentiful Omega-3 essential fatty acids. Above that is the layer including poultry, eggs, and cheese, which are eaten only about once a week. Sweets, red meat, and processed foods are placed on the top tier of the pyramid, which means they are consumed rarely or not at all. In countries like Italy, sweets like gelato are eaten in moderation. This milk-based dessert is high in protein and calcium. Other Med countries are famous for their fruit tarts: in-season fruits are converted into delicious desserts to complement the lower sections of the food pyramid.

Beverages like wine and water are shown on the side of the pyramid. The Mediterranean is a warm region, and people there drink plenty of fluids. Red wine is a cultural staple of Mediterranean cuisine. The verdict is still out on this aspect of the Med diet[5] — specifically regarding the benefits of resveratrol, a primary compound in red wine, and whether it is beneficial to heart health. If you plan on consuming a glass of red wine daily to complement the Mediterranean recipes in this book, it is best that you talk to your doctor first.

The Science Behind The Diet: Why It Works

The Mediterranean diet is ideal for weight loss for a number of key reasons:

- The lack of red meat and steak.

- The abundance of leafy green vegetables.

- Heart-healthy olive oil as a cooking medium.

- A healthy attitude toward food.

A healthy diet is more than the sum of its parts. We cannot reiterate enough than the diet is not just about food, but also about lifestyle. The mind plays an important role in our overall health and wellbeing. When you exercise daily and eat your meals mindfully as a shared experience with family and friends, you are more likely to eat healthier. You start loving yourself and your body more; as a result, you make wiser food choices and prefer putting healthy food in your body.

Another reason the diet works is due to lower consumption of red meat. In typical American fare, the high consumption of meat, which takes days to digest, leads to constipation. The abundance of whole grains, leafy green vegetables, and colorful fruits in the Med diet provides us with adequate fiber, which is very important to prevent heart disease. Fiber also encourages bowel movement and helps eliminate toxins from the body.

Plant-based diets like the Med diet also provide higher levels of antioxidants. Antioxidants fight free radicals, which are rogue molecules that can turn cancerous. Free radicals also cause premature aging in the form of age spots, wrinkles, fine lines, and gray hair. Regular consumption of antioxidant-rich foods found in the Mediterranean diet, especially nuts, seeds, and fruits, might actually help you look younger. It can also lower the risk of certain cancers.

No doubt you've heard about plenty of fad diets before, and you may be wondering what makes the Mediterranean diet any different. But far from being a trendy new fad with no scientific basis, the Med diet has been known to give consistent results. Ancel Keys, who is now known as the Father of the Med Diet, has recorded journals of data and case studies that show how the people who adopted these eating habits have gone on to lead healthier, happier, and longer lives.

Benefits of Med Diet

The Mediterranean diet can:

- Increase longevity

- Prevent asthma and allergies

- Reduce the risk of certain cancers

- Reduce the risk of type II diabetes

- Reduce depression and anxiety

- Improve mood and mental function

- Improve the look and feel of skin

- Prevent many chronic conditions

- Provide a 72% reduction in the risk of death from heart disease[6]

- Safeguard against Parkinson's disease and Alzheimer's disease

- Aid in weight loss and help in weight management

- Reduce body fat and improve metabolism

- Reduce high blood pressure

- Lower LDL (bad cholesterol) and raise HDL (good cholesterol)

- Improve heart health and artery health.

Myths And Facts About The Med Diet

Myth: The Mediterranean diet is hard to follow.

The fact is that the diet is filled with foods you can easily get in the local supermarket or farmer's market. There are no hard-to-acquire foreign foods. The diet includes plenty of foods you're already familiar with and may be eating already, like yogurt, whole grains, vegetables, nuts, and seeds — the Med diet simply changes the balance so that these foods make up the bulk of your meals. Compared to many other diets out there, the Mediterranean diet is easy to adopt because there is no deprivation. You do not eliminate any food groups. You can eat everything as long as you do so in moderation. Certain foods, like sweets and processed foods, should be eaten in limited quantities, but there is no reason that you cannot enjoy them occasionally.

Myth: I am allowed to eat anything on the diet.

All food groups are permitted in the Mediterranean diet, but it is very important to follow the Med food pyramid and to control portion size. The intake of sugary desserts and meats should be limited, and it is very important to balance the intake of food with adequate exercise and proper eating patterns. The key is to eat food mindfully and to share meals with family or friends. When you share food with other healthy, like-minded people, you are more likely to limit your portions and make health-conscious choices.

Myth: The Mediterranean diet is expensive.

The diet includes cooking meals with olive oil, seed oils, and nut oils, which can be a bit expensive compared to other cooking mediums. However, the key is to shop smart. If you take the time to plan your weekly meals properly, you can avoid waste and buy only what you need. Think about buying ingredients in bulk to get the most bang for your buck. Buy fruits and vegetables only while they are in season to get the best prices. If fresh fillets are too expensive to buy on a regular basis, you can buy tilapia, tuna, or other frozen cuts to supplement fresh fish. You can also buy a wide variety of canned and dry beans in bulk. These versatile ingredients can keep your meals interesting without breaking the bank.

Myth: The Med diet is just a fad diet.

Put simply, the Mediterranean diet works. It is not a diet, but a lifestyle. Unlike many other fad diets out there, it does not consist of eliminating any food groups, meaning that the diet is ideal for the long term and does not lead to nutritional deficiencies. You also eat a variety of foods that are proven to be heart healthy. Years of research prove that the diet can be adopted as a sustainable lifestyle that helps to maintain a healthy weight and ward off a host of diseases that are so common in the Western world.

Case Studies On The Mediterranean Diet

Many case studies[7] have shown the efficacy of the Med diet in reducing mortality and preventing cardiovascular diseases, breast cancer, type II diabetes, and hypertension. 100 or more people who followed the diet for one year with no restriction on fat intake showed a reduced incidence of each of these diseases.

The Predimed study[8]: This was a large study conducted with more than 7000 people with a high risk of cardiovascular disease. The result: Participants who were placed on a Mediterranean diet high in olives, olive oil, and nuts showed a lower incidence of cardiovascular disease.

The reversal of Metabolic Syndrome status[9]: This study showed that the traditional Mediterranean diet, with an emphasis on consuming high amount of nuts, could be a significant tool in managing Metabolic Syndrome, which is a condition responsible for several heart diseases as well as diabetes.

On weight loss[10]: A meta analysis of 16 randomized trials on the effect of the Med diet on body weight showed that Mediterranean diet resulted in greater weight loss compared to the control diet, when associated with energy restriction and physical activity.

Chapter 2: Adopting The Med Lifestyle

Once you have read through this book, you will know which foods to eat and which ones to avoid. It is a good idea to make a detailed shopping list in order to plan your weekly meals. The diet is extremely varied — you can choose from a wide range of fruits, vegetables, seafood, and more. So if you don't like shrimp, you don't need to buy it. Just go for any other seafood that is affordable and available in season.

Remember that just because the diet is called "Mediterranean" does not mean that you cannot eat Japanese, Indian, or other types of dishes. Just make sure you choose the right ingredients and prepare the food in accordance with basic Mediterranean principles.

How To Lose Weight On The Med Diet

In order to lose weight most efficiently on this diet, we recommend that you eat small but frequent meals. Do not skip any meals as it can affect your blood sugar levels and cause you to binge later. Opt for healthy "mini meals" and snacks that can provide your body with all the nutrition it needs.

Making wise choices and planning ahead is the best way to adopt the Med lifestyle. Spend some time putting together a salad with different seasonal fruits, vegetables, and nuts. Make a nice big batch and keep it in the fridge so that you always have something to snack on when you're hungry.

Use the same idea with plain vegetables. You can cut up enough for a few a days at a time; then just make sure you have a supply of healthy salad dressings to dip them in, and you have an extremely healthy, convenient snack whenever you want it. Stock up on nuts and seeds, which are full of protein and can help curb hunger between meals.

Start thinking in terms of portion sizes rather than calories. Instead of heaping up a plate with everything on the table, focus on smaller portions of a few specific items. By appreciating every dish or food item on your plate, you'll learn to enjoy and savor each portion rather than wolfing down everything that's in front of you.

More than any particular food group, the main thing to avoid is stress. Counting calories and depriving your body of needed nutrition heightens levels of cortisol, a stress hormone. Cortisol wreaks havoc on metabolism and increases the storage of fat in the abdomen, thighs, and hips.

Starting Out

We've prepared a convenient, readymade shopping list for you to begin your Mediterranean diet. Before you get started, make sure you get every family member on board. Having the support of the people you share your meals with will be key in successfully sticking to the diet.

Once everyone is informed and excited about the Med diet, go through your pantry and throw out the unhealthy food. Margarine, donuts, cookies, frozen processed foods — you don't need them anymore, and it's best to remove temptation.

Here is a list of staples to buy for your Mediterranean pantry.

Stocking Your Mediterranean Kitchen

- Olive oil, coconut oil, clarified butter. Buy a large quantity of extra virgin olive oil

- Walnuts, cashew nuts, almonds, macadamia nuts, Brazil nuts

- Seeds: flaxseeds, sunflower seeds, sesame seeds

- Vinegar: red, white, apple cider, and balsamic

• Spices: oregano, turmeric, thyme, powdered garlic, cumin, salt, onion powder, curry, sea salt, black pepper, basil, mint, dill, red chili flakes, and Mrs. Dash seasonings

• Sweetener: Throw out the refined sugar and switch to sweeteners like maple syrup, agave nectar, stevia, honey, or molasses.

• Flours: Natural gluten-free flours, arrowroot starch

• Bread: Sprouted bread, or Ezekiel bread, is available in health food stores. Look for unseasoned bread crumbs and plain croutons.

• Whole wheat pasta

• Brown rice, wild rice, basmati rice

• Polenta

• Couscous

• Bulgur

• Quinoa

• Canned tuna, salmon

• Fresh seasonal fish

• Chicken

• Canned tomatoes and tomato paste

• Red wine

• Vegetables: asparagus, artichokes, cabbage, cauliflower, eggplant, zucchini, mushrooms, onions, tomatoes, carrots, bell peppers, broccoli, spinach, leafy green vegetables, green beans

• Fruits: oranges, apples, strawberries, blueberries, raspberries, blackberries, grapes, cherries, lemons, figs, plums, dates, peaches, melons, cantaloupes, avocados

• Dairy and poultry: skim milk, Greek yogurt, cheese (parmesan, mozzarella, etc.), cage free eggs

• Condiments: honey mustard, unsweetened ketchup, vinaigrette, organic mayonnaise made with cage free eggs, tahini sauce, low sodium peanut butter

• Snacks: hummus, organic salsa, organic trail mix, almonds, sesame seeds and other nuts, unsalted kale and soy chips, wasa crackers, unsalted crackers, plain rice cakes. To make homemade hummus: blend together chickpeas, salt, garlic, lime juice and tahini

• Canned soups: organic soups for days you are too tired to cook

• Other staples: bottled garlic, stuffed olives, artichoke hearts, wild caught sardines

• Occasional Treats: dark chocolate with at least 70% cocoa

Stock your healthy Med pantry with items you can store for 3-6 months. Shop in your neighborhood organic store and select items with the USDA organic stamp of approval. Buy items in bulk or when they are on sale.

More tips to adjust to the healthy Med diet

1. Try something new once a week. This will keep things from getting mundane.

2. Drink plenty of water. Most hunger pangs are actually thirst, so keep a water bottle near you all the time. The Med diet will also give you lots of fiber, so drinking water will keep the fiber moving efficiently through your system.

3. When you're hungry, reach for something from the bottom of the food pyramid. Fruits, vegetables, whole grain breads, and other items from this layer will give you more fiber and keep you full longer.

4. Men may consume up to 1800 calories and women up to 1200 calories per day. If you want to enjoy more calories, aim to burn more calories throughout the day.

With moderate daily exercise, you can easily lose up to 2 lbs per week on the Mediterranean diet by following these meal plans and low-calorie recipes.

Weekly Diet Plan

	Breakfast	Lunch	Snack	Dinner
Day 1	Fruit and Yogurt Smoothie	Black bean salad	Hummus with vegetables	Pasta with salad
Day 2	Couscous	Grilled Salmon	Tzatziki dip with pita bread or veggies	Cabbage apple slaw with baked fish
Day 3	Omelette	Chickpea and bean soup	Fruit and nut bar	One pot turkey or chicken dish
Day 4	Oatmeal	Beans and Rice	Grilled fruit	Chicken Casserole
Day 5	Fruit and Yogurt Parfait	Vegetable wrap	Boiled eggs	Healthy bean soup with bread and salad
Day 6	Buckwheat Pancakes	Vegetable Pasta	Wholegrain toast or crackers with cheese	Grilled fish/chicken with brown rice
Day 7	Frittata	Grilled Chicken	Yogurt with fruit	Healthy Pizza

Chapter 3: Mediterranean Breakfast Recipes

Breakfast is the most important meal of the day. All the breakfast recipes included here are quick, simple, and low in calories.

1. Kickstart Your Day Berry Smoothie

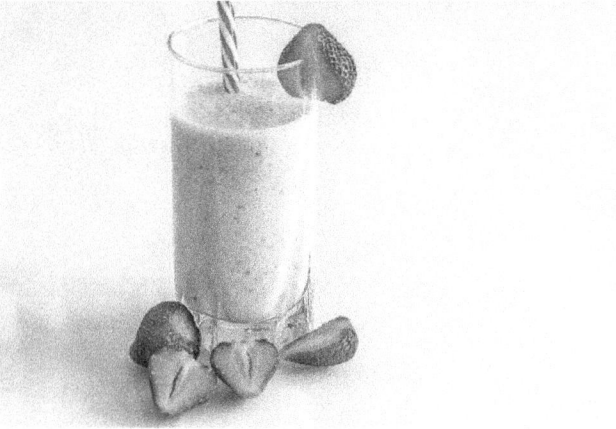

(Prep: 5 minutes. Calories: 100)

Ingredients

- 1 juicy peach
- ½ cup Greek yogurt or plain yogurt
- 1 small banana, peeled
- ⅔ cup hulled strawberries
- 1 tsp flaxseeds

Method

- Cut the peach in half, remove the pit and cube the pulp.

• Add all ingredients to a food processor.

• Blitz until the ingredients are combined.

• Serve immediately, or chill for an hour before serving.

2. Yogurt Bowl

(Prep time: 5 minutes. Calories: 364. Protein: 24g)

Ingredients

- 1 cup plain Greek yogurt
- ½ banana sliced
- 3 strawberries hulled and sliced
- ¼ cup fresh blueberries
- 2 tbsp raw local organic honey.

Method

- In a bowl, place the yogurt.
- Add the sliced banana and berries.
- Drizzle honey on top.
- Serve chilled.

Tip: Make the breakfast bowl more nutritious by sprinkling seeds and nuts on it.

3. Mediterranean Omelet

(Prep time: 10 minutes. Calories: 560. Protein: 20g)

This omelet is packed with protein and vegetables.

Ingredients

- 2 large eggs

- 2 tbsp extra virgin olive oil

- 1 medium yellow onion chopped

- 1 clove garlic minced

- 1 cup spinach chopped

- ½ medium tomato diced

- 2 tbsp skim milk

- 4 kalamata olives pitted and diced

- Salt and pepper to taste

- 3 tbsp crumbled feta cheese

- 1 tbsp chopped fresh parsley

Method

- In a frying pan, heat the oil.

- Add onions and fry till browned. Also add garlic and fry for 2 minutes.

- Add the salt, spinach and tomatoes and cook for a few minutes.

• In a bowl, whisk together egg and milk.

• Add pepper and olives to the pan and pour the egg mixture over the sautéed vegetables.

• Spread around and turn the heat up so the egg cooks quickly. You can lift the omelet a bit to allow the upper liquid layer to go underneath the cooked egg. Continue cooking till the egg is cooked.

• Fold the omelet in half. Slide onto a plate and add cheese and freshly chopped parsley. Serve warm.

4. Buckwheat Pancakes

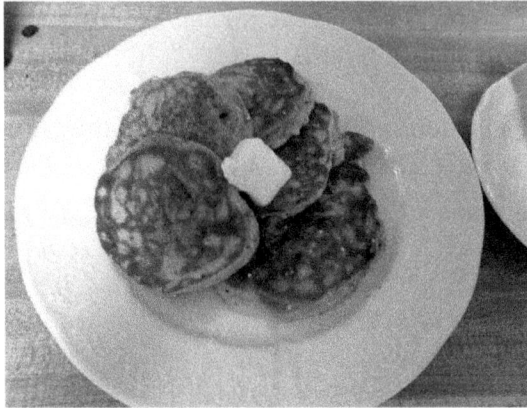

(Prep time: 20 minutes. Calories: 240. Protein: 11g. Fiber: 12g)

Buckwheat is a cereal grain and one of the healthiest foods you can have for breakfast.

Ingredients

- 1 egg

- ¼ tsp baking soda

- 1 tsp baking powder

- 1 ¼ cup buttermilk

- 1 cup buckwheat flour

- 1 ½ tsp Stevia sweetener

- ¼ tsp vanilla extract

- Pinch of salt

- 1 tbsp clarified butter (also called ghee, this is much healthier than regular butter. You can make it at home by boiling regular unsalted butter till the whey separates, and you are left with clear brown liquid on top). You can also use regular butter.

Method

• In a bowl, mix together buckwheat flour, soda, baking powder, sweetener and salt.

• In another bowl, mix all wet ingredients: buttermilk, extract, and egg. Whisk together.

• Mix the dry and wet ingredients to form a thick, smooth batter. Let it rest for 15 minutes.

• Heat a skillet and add some clarified ghee or butter.

• Pour a large spoonful of batter in the center of the skillet a few inches in diameter and less than an inch in thickness. Let the batter bubble over which indicates it is time to flip it.

• Flip the pancake and cook on both sides, pouring some more butter or ghee if needed to prevent sticking. Pancake is done once it is brown, in about 2-3 minutes.

• Repeat these steps for the remaining batter.

• Serve the pancakes warm with maple syrup, fruit or honey.

5. Breakfast Couscous

(Prep time: 18 minutes. Calories: 259. Protein: 13g)

Couscous is a popular alternative to rice and pasta, and you can have it for breakfast without piling on too many calories to your daily allowance.

Ingredients

- 1 cup uncooked whole wheat couscous
- 3 cups skim milk
- One 2" cinnamon stick
- 6 tsp brown sugar divided
- Pinch of salt
- 4 tsp butter divided
- ¼ cup raisins and currants
- ½ cup dried apricots

Method

- In a medium pan, combine milk and cinnamon and boil for 3 minutes, stirring continuously.
- Remove from heat; add the dried fruits, couscous, currants and salt and 4 tsp of brown sugar to the pan. Mix well. Cover and keep aside for 15 minutes.
- Pour into 4 serving bowls and add 1 tsp butter and ½ tsp brown sugar on top of each bowl. Stir and serve immediately.

6. Simple Mediterranean Breakfast a la Roma

(Prep time: 10 minutes. Calories: 425. Protein: 12g)

This is a simple Roman breakfast eaten in the summer, when the tomatoes are full of rich flavors.

Ingredients

- 50g fresh ricotta cheese

- 2 boiled or poached eggs

- 1 slice sourdough rye bread

- 2-3 slices of fresh Roma tomatoes

- 1-2 tsp olive oil

- Sea salt and fresh black pepper to taste

Method

• Spread the ricotta on the bread, top with eggs. On the plate, place the assembled bread next to tomato wedges. Drizzle olive oil and season with salt and pepper.

7. Oatmeal With Fruits And Nuts

(Prep time: 5 minutes. Calories: 150 with water, or 230 if you use skim milk.)

Breakfast cannot get any simpler than this.

Ingredients

- ½ cup oats (will cook to 1 cup)

- 1 cup skim milk or water

- ¼ tsp cinnamon

- 1 chopped apple

- Handful of raisins

- ¼ cup dried cranberries

- Assorted nuts, blanched and slivered to sprinkle on top

- ½ tsp brown sugar, molasses, Stevia or honey (optional)

Method

- Cook the oats as per instructions, and add remaining ingredients.

- Add seasonal fruits and nuts to enhance the flavor of the oatmeal. You can add blueberries, strawberries and maple syrup for a classic combination.

8. Fruit And Yogurt Parfait With Granola

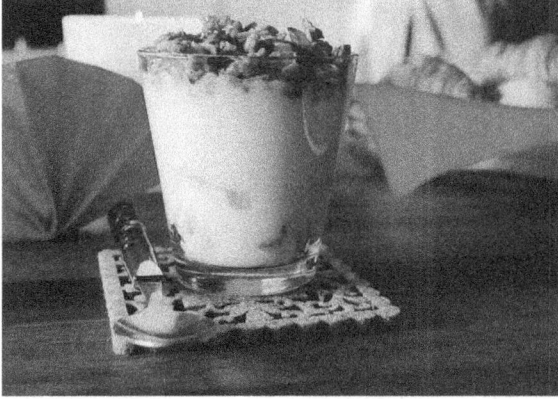

(Prep time: 5 minutes. Calories: 200.)

Another simple breakfast for the weight watchers on the Med diet, this is a quick and easy recipe that is tasty, healthy and crunchy.

Ingredients

- 1 cup low fat plain Greek yogurt
- 1 tsp honey
- ¼ cup granola cereal
- Fresh or frozen fruits

Method

- Mix yogurt and honey. Add the fruit and sprinkle granola on top.

Tip: Do not stir the granola into the mixture to keep it crispy.

9. Italian Omelet

(Prep time: 25 minutes. Calories: 450)

This is a delicious breakfast served in Italy.

Ingredients

- 1 cup sliced mushrooms and zucchini

- 3 tbsp olive oil divided

- 4 eggs

- 3 tbsp water

- Salt and pepper

- ½ cup mozzarella

- For the sauce: 1 tbsp olive oil, 1 chopped medium tomato, 2 tbsp chopped parsley, 1 clove garlic, ½ tsp basil, pinch of salt.

Method

- In a skillet, heat some olive oil and add the zucchini and mushrooms. Sauté until brown. Keep them aside (warm).

- In a bowl, whisk together eggs, water, salt and pepper. Heat the skillet and add remaining oil. Add the beaten eggs. Cook for a few minutes. As the eggs cook, push the uncooked portion beneath, and let the top part set. One the eggs are cooked, add the vegetables over one side and sprinkle mozzarella cheese. Fold the other half of the egg over the filling. Remove the eggs on a plate.

- To make the sauce, heat the oil. Add tomatoes, garlic, basil and parsley. Cook until heated through.

- Serve the sauce with the omelet.

10. Healthy Porridge With Rolled Oats

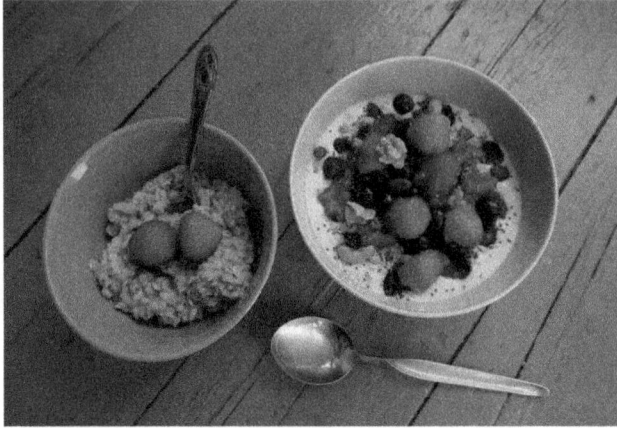

(Prep time: 5 minutes. Calories: 223)

This porridge contains oats and yogurt. It is a cold porridge that is great for breakfast or for an afternoon snack. Make a larger batch and store the porridge in the fridge for up to 4 days.

Ingredients

- 1 cup low fat plain yogurt mixed with ½ 36bsp. honey, or 1 cup vanilla flavored yogurt

- ¼ cup rolled oats

- 1 tbsp rye flakes

- Plums, sliced bananas, ground cinnamon and some more yogurt to serve.

Method

- Mix oats and rye flakes with yogurt and let stand overnight in the refrigerator.

• In the morning, serve with plums, cinnamon, bananas and yogurt and drizzle some more honey on top.

Chapter 4: Mediterranean Lunch Recipes

Did you know that the Med diet is also called the "anti-cancer diet?"[11] In this chapter, we will be covering easy lunch recipes that won't take too much of your time and will provide an abundant supply of antioxidants. The main ingredients are healthy grains, seasonal vegetables, and lean meat. Enjoy!

1. Polenta

(Prep time: 15 minutes. Calories: 112. Protein: 5g)

Serve this polenta dish with your favorite bread or soup, or enjoy it alone.

Ingredients

- ½ cup cornmeal or yellow polenta
- 1 cup skim milk
- 2 cups homemade stock or water
- 1 cup cheese
- 1-2 tbsp butter (optional)

Method

- Bring water/stock and milk to a boil.
- Add the polenta and whisk. Stir continuously.
- Polenta will take about 10 minutes to cook. The consistency should resemble mashed potatoes.
- Remove from heat. Add cheese.
- Cover and keep for 5 minutes.

• Serve warm.

2. Moroccan Chickpea Soup

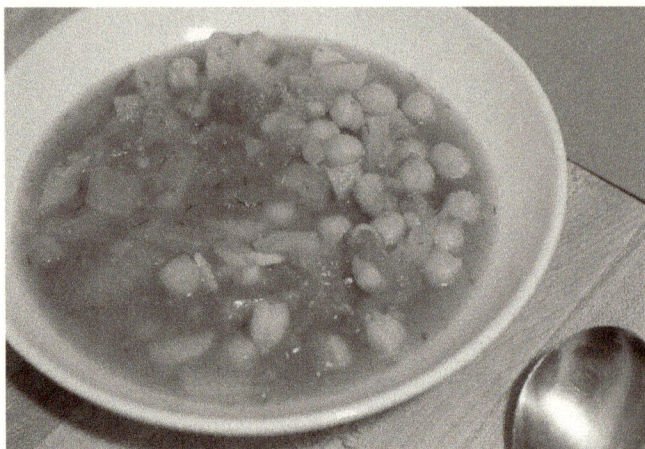

(Prep time: 20 minutes. Calories: 107)

This is a hearty soup recipe perfect for cold days. You can make a large batch and keep it in the refrigerator for up to 3 days. Pack it in an airtight container and take it to work.

Ingredients

- 2 tsp olive oil

- 1 medium onion, chopped

- 2 medium carrots, diced

- 2 celery sticks, cleaned and diced

- 2 cans of chickpeas rinsed

- 1 can of low sodium tomatoes

- 2 crushed garlic cloves

- 2 tsp Moroccan seasoning

- 2 cups low sodium vegetable or chicken stock

- 1 cup water

- Fresh coriander leaves, chopped (optional)

- Fresh low fat yogurt (optional)

- Black pepper to taste

Method

- In a large saucepan, heat the oil and add the chopped veggies. Cover and cook for 3 minutes until vegetables are soft.

- Add garlic and fry for a minute.

- Add the chickpeas, tomatoes, stock and water. Bring the mixture to a boil, then cover and simmer for up to 10 minutes.

- Remove half the soup in a bowl and cool. Pour this half in a blender and blend until creamy. Return the creamy soup to the remaining soup in the pan. Heat over medium heat for 2-3 minutes.

- Ladle into bowls and serve with yogurt (optional), and garnish with freshly chopped cilantro or coriander leaves.

3. Bean And Salmon Stir Fry

(Prep time: 10 minutes. Calories: 127)

Seafood and Chinese food lovers will love this bean and salmon stir fry recipe. Serve with brown rice for a filling and healthy meal.

Ingredients

- ¼ cup water

- 2 tbsp each rice vinegar and black bean garlic sauce.

- 1 tbsp dry sherry

- 2 tbsp cornflour

- 1 tbsp olive oil

- 500g salmon chopped into small cubes

- 2 cups mung sprouts

- 1 bunch sliced scallions.

Method

- In a small bowl, mix water, cornflour, vinegar, bean garlic sauce and sherry.

- In a large skillet, heat the oil and add the salmon cubes. Fry the pieces until browned. Add the mung bean sprouts, scallions and the bean garlic sauce mixture. Stir to coat the salmon pieces.

- Cook for 2-3 minutes until the sprouts are tender.

- Serve with sautéed veggies or brown rice.

4. Easy Red Cabbage And Walnut Slaw

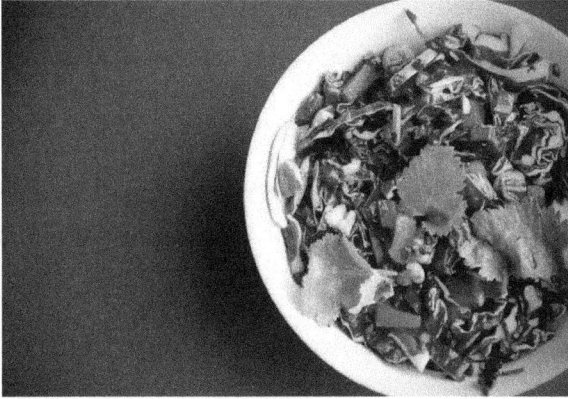

(Prep time: 10 minutes. Calories: 150)

This delicious, light slaw is an ideal alternative to traditional coleslaw.

Ingredients

- ½ red cabbage sliced thin

- 1 large apple, cored, peeled and grated

- 1 finely chopped shallot

- 2 tbsp apple cider vinegar or red wine vinegar

- 2 tbsp raisins

- Handful of walnuts, chopped

- 2 tbsp each walnut oil and olive oil

- Salt and pepper to taste

- Cilantro sprigs (optional)

Method

• In a bowl, mix the shallot and vinegar and allow the mixture to infuse for 5 minutes.

• Add the oils, seasonings and cabbage. Mix together.

• Add the grated apple and combine.

• Add the raisins and nuts and mix well. You can allow the salad to rest for half an hour or eat immediately. Garnish with cilantro.

• Variation: Add finely chopped tomatoes in place of apple as shown in image above.

5. Easy Shrimp & Chicken Paella

(Prep time: 30 minutes. Calories: 332)

Paella is a Spanish rice dish with chicken or seafood. Your family will love its distinctive flavor and bright colors. The best part is that this dish contains turmeric, an extremely healthy spice with anti-cancer[12] properties.

Ingredients

- 1 tbsp olive oil

- 1 chopped onion

- 2 red bell peppers, sliced

- 6 oz chicken sausages, cubed

- 0.5 lb chicken breasts, cubed

- 3 cups cooked brown rice

- 1 ½ cups frozen peas (thawed)

- 3 garlic cloves crushed

- 3 tsp lemon juice

- 2 tsp each turmeric and coriander powders

- 12 oz small frozen shrimp, peeled

Method

- In a skillet, heat the oil and add onions, peppers, chicken breast cubes and sausage. Fry for a minute then cover and cook for 3-4 minutes until the sausage and chicken breast is cooked thoroughly.

• In a bowl, add rice, lemon juice, peas, garlic, turmeric and coriander powders. Mix well.

• Add the rice mixture to the skillet with chicken. Place the shrimp on top of the rice and cover and cook on low heat until shrimp are cooked through, about 3 minutes.

6. Colorful Vegetable Lentil Medley

(Prep time: 25 minutes. Calories: 300. Protein: 22g)

This is a vegetarian dish with lentils and nutritious veggies. It's a delicious, high-protein recipe that still has very few calories.

Ingredients

- 2 cups vegetable broth

- 1 cup water

- 1 cup lentils, washed

- 3-4 cloves of garlic, crushed

- A pinch of salt, pepper and oregano each

- 6 cups veggies — cubed, sliced or chopped: broccoli, bell peppers, carrots, squash and onions

- 2 tbsp finely chopped mint

- 2 oz crumbled goat cheese

- For the dressing: 1 tbsp Dijon mustard, 2 tbsp olive oil, 1 tsp lemon juice

Method

- In a large pot, heat the stock and water. Add the lentils, salt, pepper, garlic, and oregano and bring to a boil. Reduce heat and simmer for 20 minutes.

- In a steamer, cook all vegetables until tender with a bit of crunch.

- Whisk together the ingredients for the dressing.

• In a large bowl, place the cooked lentils, vegetables, and dressing. Toss until coated.

• Add the crumbled cheese on top and serve.

7. Greek Plaki (Fishy Vegetable Bake)

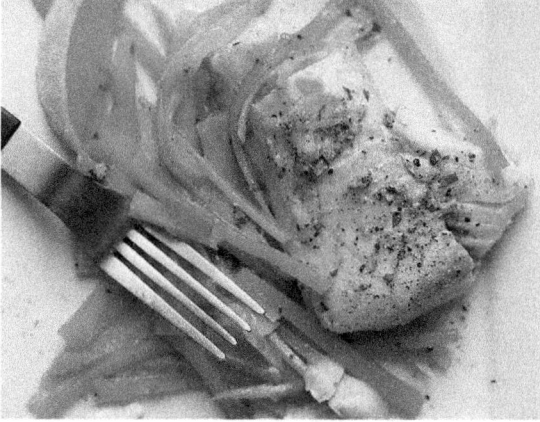

(Prep time: 30 minutes. Calories: 430)

This is a classic Greek dish that can be eaten hot or cold.

Ingredients

- 3 tbsp olive oil

- 2 medium onions, chopped

- 2 cloves garlic, crushed

- 1 celery stick, cubed

- 2 carrots, sliced

- ¼ cup vegetable stock or water

- ¼ cup white wine

- 2 tomatoes chopped

- 600g firm fish (like cod) cut into steaks or fillet

- 10-12 olives, chopped

- 3 slices of lemon

- Salt, pepper and oregano

Method

- Preheat oven to 350 degrees.

- In a pan, soften onions in olive oil for a few minutes. Add garlic, vegetables, water/stock and wine. Simmer for 5-7 minutes until vegetables are tender. Add tomatoes and oregano and cook for 2-3 minutes more.

- In an oven proof dish, lay the fillets and pour the sauce over them. Scatter the olives over them and add three lemon slices evenly. Cover with an aluminum foil and bake 20 minutes or until the fish flakes when prodded with knife.

- Cool for at least five minutes before serving.

8. Easy Sicilian Eggplant Caponata (Stew)

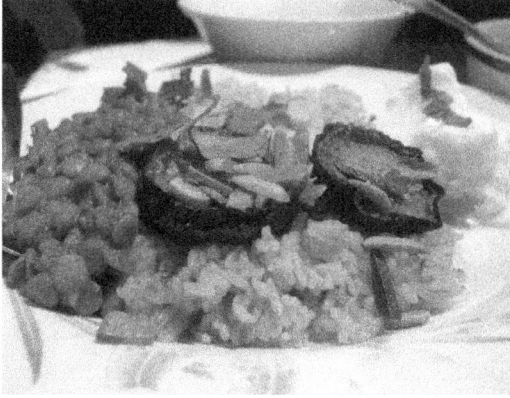

(Prep time: 30 minutes. Calories: 110)

This dish has a variety of flavors and textures. It has soft eggplant, fragrant and crunchy pine nuts, and fruity tomatoes accompanied by earthy basil. Serve it with brown rice.

Ingredients

- 2 eggplants, diced

- 1 medium onion, sliced

- 4 celery sticks, sliced

- 4-5 tomatoes, chopped

- 4 tbsp olive oil

- 12 black olives, chopped

- 2 tbsp red wine vinegar

- 1 tbsp acacia honey

- 2 tbsp basil or parsley, chopped

- 2 tbsp roasted pine nuts, crushed

- 2 tbsp capers

- Salt and pepper

Method

- Heat olive oil in a heavy bottomed skillet. Add onions and brown them.

- Add celery and eggplants and cook for 10 minutes, stirring occasionally to prevent the vegetables from sticking to the bottom or burning.

- Add tomatoes, honey, capers, olives, and wine vinegar. Cover and cook for 10-12 minutes.

- Before serving, add the parsley or basil and chopped nuts.

9. Grilled Salmon With Herbs

(Prep time: 30 minutes. Calories: 367)

Ingredients

- 450g salmon fillet

- 2 lemon slices

- 20-30 sprigs of fresh herbs like rosemary, thyme, sage, parsley, etc. chopped and divided into 2 batches

- 1 clove garlic, crushed

- 1 tbsp Dijon mustard

Method

- Fire the grill to medium high.

- On a rimless baking sheet, add two layers of heavy duty aluminium foil. Arrange lemon slices in the center of the foil. Add the sprigs of herbs on the slices.

- Crush the garlic with salt. Mix the paste of garlic and salt with 2 tbsp of chopped herbs.

- Spread the mixture on both sides of the fillets.

- Place the salmon over the herb stack. Pick up the foil off the baking sheet and slide it on the grill keeping the salmon, lemon and herbs intact.

- Close the grill and grill the fish on medium high for 18-20 minutes.

- Serve with rice, seasonal grilled vegetables or roasted baby potatoes.

10.   Chicken Scaloppine With Lemon Basil Sauce
(Prep time: 20 minutes. Calories: 180)

Don't let the name of this dish intimidate you — it's less complicated than it sounds!

Ingredients

- 1 tbsp olive oil

- ½ cup dry white wine

- ½ cup low sodium chicken broth

- 4 chicken breasts (pound them first to flatten)

- 2 tbsp each lemon juice and capers, drained

- ½ tsp each Worcestershire sauce and ground pepper

- ½ cup parsley chopped

Method

- Heat oil in a non-stick skillet and add wine and broth. Bring to a boil.

- Add chicken and cover. Cook for about 6-8 minutes.

- Remove the chicken from the skillet and keep it covered.

- Continue cooking the leftover sauce in the skillet. Add lemon juice, capers, Worcestershire sauce and pepper. Return the chicken to the sauce and add parsley. Heat through.

- Variation: Add an assortment of colorful vegetables to this recipe to get antioxidants and phytochemicals. Serve as is or with brown rice.

11.   Corn Ham Risotto

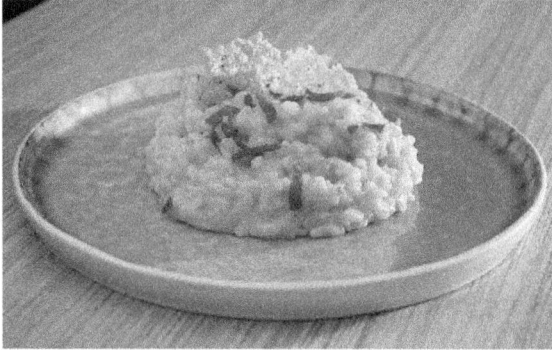

(Prep time: 30 minutes. Calories: 584)

Ingredients

- 2 tbsp olive oil

- 2 cloves of garlic, crushed

- 1 chopped shallot

- 1 ½ cup Arborio rice

- Salt and pepper to taste

- ¾ cup dry white wine

- 4 cups stock (chicken or vegetable) or water

- 2 cups corn kernels

- 8 oz shredded smoked ham

- 4 oz cheese

- ½ cup chives, chopped (leave some for garnish)

Method

- In a large sauce pan, heat the oil. Add garlic and shallots. Cook for several minutes.

- Add the rice and fry briefly.

- Add wine and stir. Cook for 1-2 minutes until liquid is absorbed.

- Season with salt and pepper.

- Add stock little at a time and cook for 5 minutes. If the rice appears dry, add remaining stock.

- Add the corn and cook until corn becomes tender. Then, add the ham.

- Stir in the cheese until melted.

- Add chives. Add salt and pepper to taste.

- Serve with more cheese and chives on top.

12. Pasta With Zucchini And Smoked Mozzarella

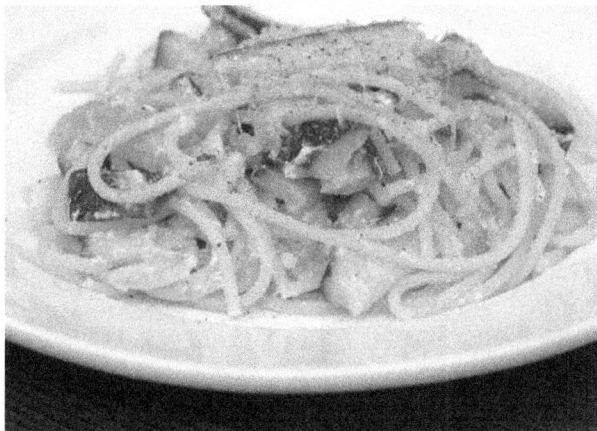

(Prep time: 30 minutes. Calories: 500)

Ingredients

- 2 tbsp butter

- 2 tbsp extra virgin olive oil

- 3 thinly sliced bell pepper

- 1 sliced onion

- 2 medium zucchini cut into ½" slices

- Salt and pepper to taste

- 12 oz pasta of your choice

- 4 oz smoked mozzarella

- ½ cup chopped basil divided for garnish

Method

- Cook pasta according to package instruction. Drain but reserve one cup water.

- In the meanwhile, heat a large sauce pan. Add oil and butter.

• Fry onions, pepper and zucchini until onions and peppers are softened and zucchini is crispy.

• Add the cheese, pasta and one cup of cooking water. Toss to coat the pasta well. Add basil and mix well.

• Add salt and pepper.

• If pasta looks dry, add some water to increase sauce.

• Serve hot, garnished with some more cheese and basil leaves.

13. Flavorful Linguine With Brussels Sprouts

(Prep time: 30 minutes. Calories: 407)

Ingredients

- 1 box linguine

- 2 tbsp olive oil

- Salt and pepper to taste

- 6 slices thick-cut pancetta or bacon

- 1 chopped medium onion

- 1 lb brussel sprouts

- 2 cloves garlic

- 3 oz cheese (parmesan or mozzarella)

- ⅓ cup dry white wine

Method

- Cook the pasta according to box instructions. Drain and set aside. Reserve one cup of cooking water.

- In a pan, heat the oil. Add garlic and onions. Fry until the onions are brown.

- Add the brussel sprouts and sauté until the sprouts turn bright green.

- Add the wine and stir until the liquid is absorbed.

- Add pasta, cheese, cooking water, salt and pepper. Mix well.

- Heat until the cheese has melted and the pasta is creamy.

- Serve with grated cheese.

14. One Pot Chicken Pasta
(Prep time: 30 minutes. Calories: 500)

Ingredients

- 1 box pasta
- 1 tbsp olive oil
- 1 lb chicken cut into bite-sized pieces
- 1 tbsp all-purpose seasoning mix
- Salt and pepper
- 3 cloves garlic
- 1 can of sun-dried tomatoes, drained and chopped
- 1 ½ cups each of mozzarella cheese and whole milk
- ½ cup half and half
- ½ cup chicken broth
- 2 cups spinach leaves

Method

- Cook pasta according to instructions. Drain and set aside.
- In a skillet, add oil and put on medium heat.
- Sauté the chicken and season it. Cook until tender.
- Add the garlic and chopped sun-dried tomatoes.
- Add milk, broth, half and half and cheese. Cook until the sauce thickens.

• Add the pasta and spinach leaves. Cook until the leaves start to cook down. If the pasta seems dry, add some more water, milk or broth.

15. Easy Avocado Bean Salad

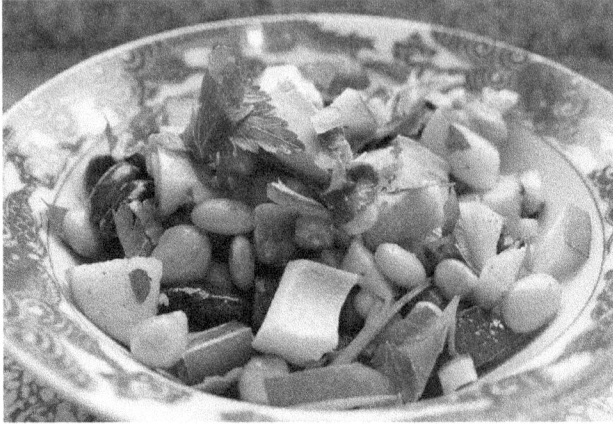

(Prep time: 20 minutes. Calories: 283)

Ingredients

- 2 large avocados, peeled, pitted and cubed

- ½ cup each chopped red bell pepper and green bell pepper

- 1 can of your choice of beans (pinto, red, etc.), washed and drained

- Large head of romaine lettuce

- For the dressing: ½ cup each olive oil and rice wine vinegar, 2 tsp each parsley and coriander, 2 tbsp honey, ½ tsp black pepper

Method

- Combine bell pepper, avocado and beans in a bowl.

- In another bowl, whisk together the dressing ingredients. Leave half of parsley for garnishing. Mix the bean mixture with the dressing to coat evenly.

• Arrange the salad over the lettuce leaves. Sprinkle leftover parsley to garnish. Serve immediately.

Chapter 5: Mediterranean Dinner Recipes

The dinner recipes included here typically take a maximum of 30 minutes to prepare, and all are nutritious and healthy. Enjoy!

1.   Creamy Vegetable Fettuccine

(Prep time: 30 minutes. Calories: 312)

Ingredients

- 8 oz fettuccine pasta

- 1 cup each sliced mushrooms, sliced red bell peppers, sliced green bell peppers and broccoli florets

- 2 tsp olive oil

- 1 tsp butter.

- 1 tbsp all purpose flour

- 2 cloves garlic crushed

- Parmesan cheese (to taste)

- 2 oz light cream cheese

- 2 oz crumbled gorgonzola cheese

- Salt and pepper

- 1 ¼ cups fat-free milk

Method

- Cook pasta according to directions.

- Steam all veggies until tender.

• In a large saucepan, heat the oil. Add crushed garlic. Let garlic brown. Then add flour and stir quickly. If desired, you can also add a teaspoon of butter.

• Add milk, cream cheese and gorgonzola cheeses. Stir and continue heating until the cheeses melt.

• Once sauce thickens, remove from heat. Now add the pasta and mix well. Add the vegetables and toss until mixed well.

• Top with grated parmesan and pepper.

2.   Spinach and Sun-Dried Tomato Pizza

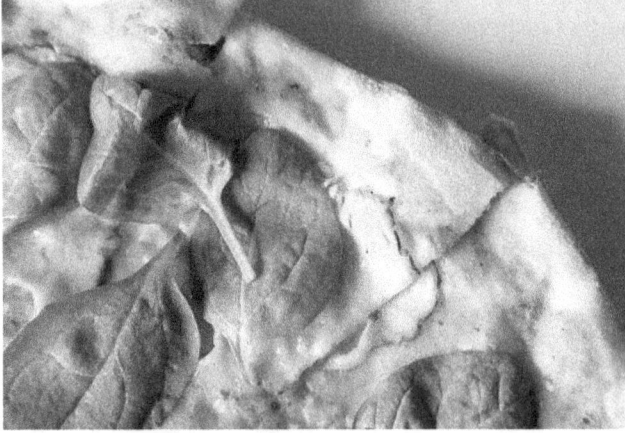

(Prep time: 25 minutes. Calories: 281 per slice)

Ingredients

- ½ cup dry packed sun-dried tomatoes

- 2 tbsp fresh basil

- 3 tbsp parmesan cheese

- ⅓ cup tomato juice

- 1 ready-to-use pizza dough base

- 1 tsp olive oil

- 2 cloves garlic

- 1 tbsp balsamic vinegar

- 2 tbsp tomato paste

- 2 cups fresh spinach leaves

Method

• Pour hot water on the sun-dried tomatoes and let them soak for 10 minutes.

• To prepare pesto: blend the tomatoes, tomato juice, tomato paste, basil, vinegar, olive oil, garlic and parmesan cheese.

• To assemble the pizza, spread the sauce on the pizza base. Top it with spinach leaves and sprinkle mozzarella on top.

• Bake according to directions until crust is cooked and cheese melts.

3.   Greek Burgers

(Prep time: 20 minutes. Calories: 338)

Ingredients

- 1 lb ground beef

- 1 tsp oregano

- ¼ tsp black pepper

- 1 tbsp garlic

- 2 tbsp red onions, minced

- 1 oz crumbled feta cheese

- 4 whole wheat hamburger buns

Method

- Preheat grill.

- To make patties: combine the beef, spices, garlic, onions and form into 8 patties. Divide the cheese evenly over 4 of the patties. Top with remaining patties. Pinch the edges to seal.

- Grill the patties. Flip midway through cooking. Leave the patties on the heat for approximately 10-12 minutes. Do not overcook.

- Assemble the burger with tomato and cucumber slices.

4.   Parmesan Garlic Salmon

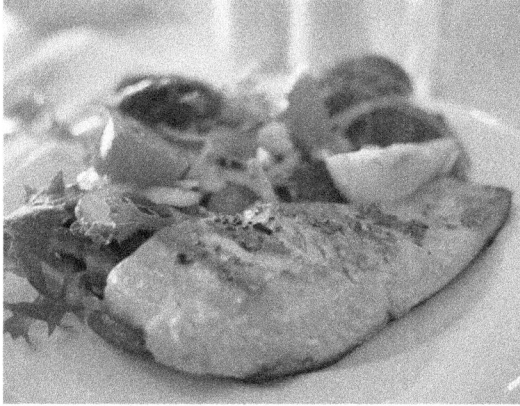

(Prep time: 20 minutes. Calories: 318)

Ingredients

- 1 lb salmon

- 1 clove minced garlic

- ½ tsp Worcestershire sauce

- ⅓ cup mayonnaise

- 3 tbsp grated parmesan cheese

- 3 tbsp chopped onions or chives

Method

- Wash the fish fillets. Pat them dry.

- To make the sauce: mix garlic, Worcestershire sauce, mayo, onions and cheese.

- Spread the sauce evenly over the fish fillets. Place the fillet on a baking dish lined with butter paper.

- Bake for 15 minutes at 450 degrees.

- Serve with a side of steamed broccoli and other vegetables.

5. Black Bean and Corn Pita Pockets

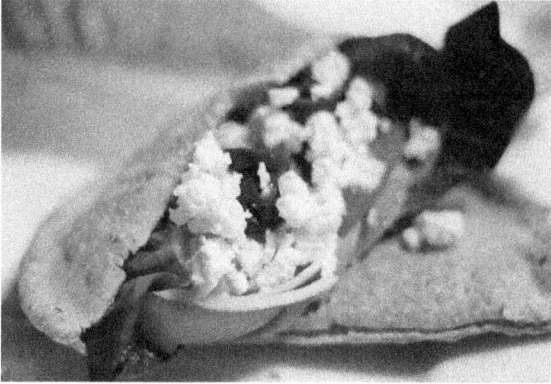

(Prep time: 15 minutes. Calories: 430)

Ingredients

- 1 can low sodium black beans, drained and rinsed

- 1 cup frozen corn (thawed)

- 1 cup low sodium canned tomatoes or fresh chopped tomatoes

- 1 chopped avocado

- 1 tsp chopped parsley

- Salt and pepper to taste

- ⅓ cup shredded mozzarella

- 2 tsp lemon juice

- 1 tsp chili powder

- 4 pita pockets made with whole wheat

Method

• In a bowl, combine beans, corn, tomatoes, avocado, parsley, lemon juice, chili powder, salt and pepper.

• Cut pita bread in half to form pockets. Fill each pocket with the bean mixture. Add cheese and parsley on top. Serve.

6.   Chicken Tortas

(Prep time: 15 minutes. Calories: 383)

Ingredients

- 2 cups of boiled and shredded chicken
- 1 tsp chili powder
- 2 cups fresh salsa
- 2 cups shredded lettuce
- 4 thin slices of white onions
- ½ cup grated cheese (feta or Monterey jack)
- 2 sliced radishes
- 1 avocado, chopped
- 1 large roll of French bread, cut in half

Method

- In a bowl, mix together the chicken, chili powder, and salsa.
- In another bowl, combine the vegetables (lettuce, onions, cheese and radishes).
- Evenly spoon the chicken and lettuce mixtures inside the bread. Top with fresh salsa and serve.

7.   Healthy Gyro

(Prep time: 25 minutes. Calories: 500)

Gyros are a Greek dish made with rotisserie meat and served inside pita pockets.

Ingredients

- 1 cup sliced onion

- 2 cups each sliced green and red bell peppers

- 1 tbsp lemon juice

- 1 tbsp olive oil

- ½ lb turkey or chicken, cut in strips

- 1 medium apple, cored and sliced

- 6 whole wheat pita pockets

- ½ cup Greek low fat yogurt

Method

- In a skillet, heat oil. Add the onion, salt, lemon juice and bell peppers. Sauté until brown and crisp.

- Stir in the chicken or turkey and sauté until the meat is cooked.

- Remove from heat. Add the apple slices.

- Beat the yogurt with a fork until liquid.

- To assemble the gyro: add the apple-meat mixture to the pita and fold. Add the yogurt on top. Serve warm.

8.   One Pot Turkey Dinner

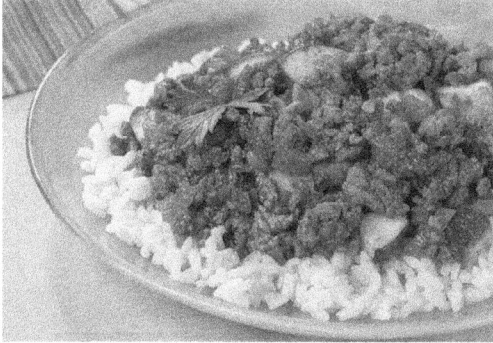

(Prep time: 30 minutes. Calories: 286)

Ingredients

- ¾ lb ground turkey

- 1 medium onion, chopped

- 2 medium zucchini, sliced

- 3 tomatoes, chopped

- 3 tbsp tomato paste

- Olive oil

- 1 tsp each oregano, thyme, basil and garlic powders

- Salt and pepper

Method

- In a pan, add olive oil and heat.

- Add the ground turkey and onions. Fry until onions are brown and soft, about 10 minutes.

- Add the remaining ingredients and simmer for 10 minutes.

- Add zucchini and cook for 5 minutes more.

- Serve with salad, white rice or brown rice.

9. Lemon Chicken with Herbs and Vegetables

(Prep time: 30 minutes. Calories: 400)

Ingredients

- ½ lb small red potatoes, cubed

- 1 ½ cups baby carrots

- 1 cup green beans, trimmed

- 2 boneless, skinless chicken breasts, halved

- 1 tbsp olive oil

- ½ cup lemon juice

- 2 tbsp honey

- 1 tbsp chopped fresh rosemary or 1 tsp dried rosemary

- 1 tsp lemon zest

- Salt and pepper to taste

Method

- Cook potatoes, carrots and beans in boiling water for 8 minutes. Drain the water and set the veggies aside.

- In a medium skillet, heat olive oil and add the chicken breasts. Cook each breast for 3-4 minutes on either side.

- Add the boiled vegetables and remaining ingredients except lemon juice to the skillet. Cover and cook for 5 minutes.

- Turn off heat. Taste test and adjust seasonings to your preference. Add lemon juice and serve with a crisp green salad.

10.   Spaghetti With Turkey Sauce
(Prep time: 30 minutes. Calories: 346)

Ingredients

- 1 lb spaghetti

- 2 cloves garlic, crushed

- Salt and pepper

- 1 tsp dried oregano

- 1 cup chopped onions

- 2 cans diced tomatoes (keep the juice)

- 1 green bell pepper chopped

- ¾ lb ground turkey

- 1-2 tbsp olive oil

Method

- Cook spaghetti according to instructions. Drain.

- Heat oil in a skillet and cook turkey for 5-7 minutes. Drain fat.

- Add bell peppers, onions, oregano and tomatoes including juice. Add salt and pepper. Cover and cook the sauce for 15 minutes, stirring occasionally.

- Pour the turkey sauce over the spaghetti and serve warm.

11.   Vegetables Wraps

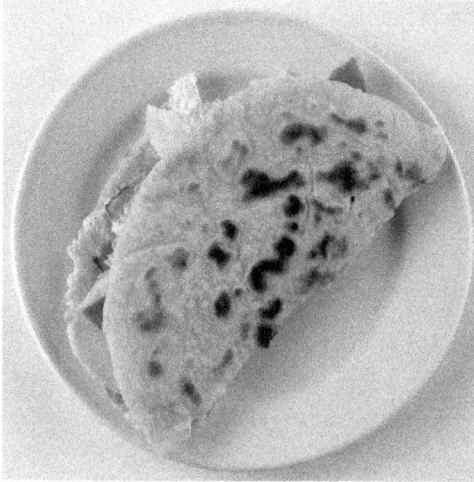

(Prep time: 20 minutes. Calories: 128)

Ingredients

- Four 7" wheat wraps

- 8 tbsp low fat cream cheese

- 2 cups shredded lettuce

- 1 cup shredded spinach

- 1 cup chopped tomato

- ½ cup mixed red, yellow and green bell peppers, chopped

- ½ cup chopped cucumber

- ¼ cup chopped chiles

- ¼ cup chopped olives

Method

- Spread cream cheese over each wrap.

- Add the vegetables over half the wrap.

- Fold and roll tightly to enclose filling. Serve.

12. Falafel

(Prep time: 30 minutes. Calories: 333)

Ingredients

- 1 can chickpeas, drained and washed

- 1 onion, chopped

- 1 garlic clove, crushed

- 1 tsp each cumin and coriander powder

- 1 tsp baking powder

- Salt and pepper to taste

- 1 egg

- Olive oil

Method

- Mash chickpeas with a masher.

- Mix all ingredients to form a sticky dough.

- Take some oil on your hands and shape the mixture into patties.

- Heat oil and fry each falafel until brown.

- Drain the falafels on a paper towel.

- Serve with ketchup, cucumber-mint yogurt dip, rice or in pita pockets.

13.   Baked Fish and Rice

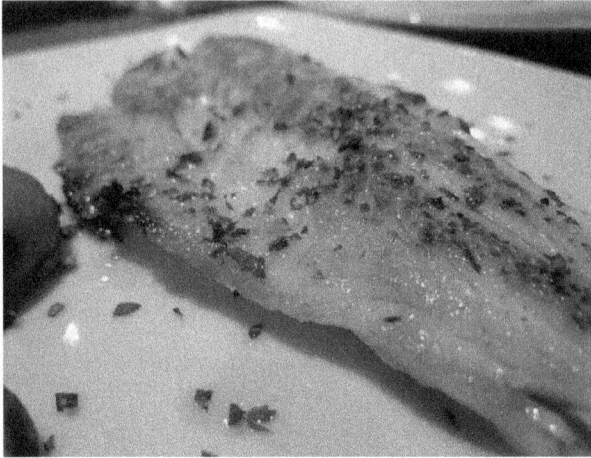

(Prep time: 25 minutes. Calories: 392)

Ingredients

- 2 tbsp olive oil

- 1 chopped onion

- 2 eggs

- 1 cup milk

- 1 cup corn kernels (or 1 cup peas)

- 1 tbsp all-purpose flour

- ¼ cup grated low fat cheese

- 2 small tins of tuna, drained and rinsed

- Salt and pepper to taste

- 4 small cups of cooked rice (or use leftovers from another dish)

Method

- Preheat oven to 350 degrees.

- In a saucepan, heat oil. Add onions and corn or peas. Cook until veggies are tender.

- Stir in the flour and mix. Remove pan from heat and slowly add in milk, whisking continuously to prevent lumps.

- Return the pan to heat and continue cooking until the sauce thickens. Turn off heat. Break the eggs into the pan and add the cheese. Mix well.

- Add tuna, salt and pepper. Add the rice. Mix.

- Prepare a casserole baking dish by applying some butter and pour in the rice mixture.

- Bake at 350 degrees for 15 minutes.

14.   Easy Couscous

(Prep time: 10 minutes. Calories: 112)

Ingredients

- 1 cube of chicken or beef bouillon, or powdered soup mix

- 1 cup water

- 1 cup couscous

Method

- Boil the water and dissolve the soup mix or bouillon cube in it.

- Pour the boiling stock cube on couscous in another bowl.

- Fluff with a fork and mix well. Cover and set aside for 10 minutes. Fluff again. Serve hot.

15.   Chunky Vegetable Soup

(Prep time: 30 minutes. Calories: 333)

Ingredients

- 2 tsp olive oil

- 1 chopped onion

- 4 cups chicken broth

- 1 ½ cups canned tomatoes

- 1 tsp each dried basil and oregano

- 1 tbsp dried parsley

- 2 bay leaves

- 2 carrots, chopped

- 2 potatoes or sweet potatoes, diced

- 2 celery stalks, diced

- 1 can kidney beans, drained and rinsed

Method

- Heat oil in a large pot.

- Add onions and brown.

- Add broth, tomatoes, basil, oregano, parsley, potatoes, celery and carrots and boil the mixture. Turn the heat down and simmer for 15 minutes until vegetables are tender.

• Add the beans and cook until heated through, about another 3 minutes. Season with salt and pepper. Serve hot with rice or bread.

Note: if you are using canned condensed broth, dilute it with a cup of water.

16.   Black Bean Salad with Avocado Lime Dressing

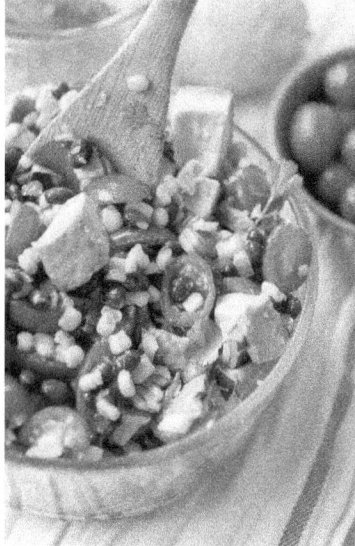

(Prep time: 10 minutes. Calories: 125)

Ingredients

- 2 cans black beans, washed

- 1 avocado, mashed

- ½ cup chopped cilantro

- 2 tbsp lime juice

- 4 cups chopped romaine lettuce

- 1 cup chopped grape tomatoes

- 1 cup frozen corn (thawed)

- 1 chopped red bell pepper

- ½ cup toasted seeds or nuts (pumpkin, pine nuts, etc.)

Method

• Whisk together cilantro, avocado and lime juice.

• Add the beans, lettuce, bell pepper and tomatoes. Toss to coat well.

• Add the corn and nuts/seeds. Mix well and serve chilled.

17.   Chicken Macaroni Casserole

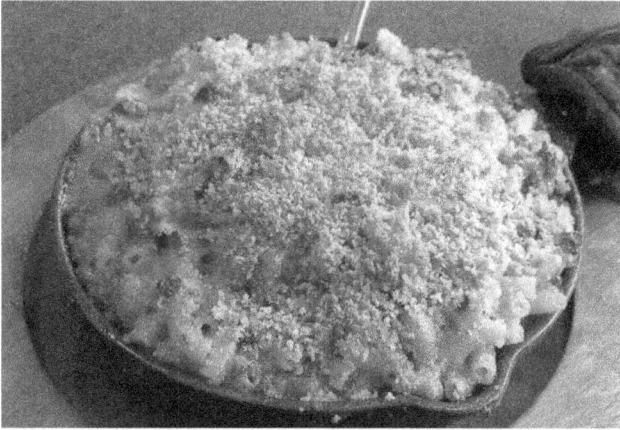

(Prep time: 25 minutes. Calories: 479)

Ingredients

- ½ lb chicken, cooked and shredded

- ½ cup chopped onions

- ½ cup milk

- 2 cans of cream of chicken soup

- Salt and pepper to taste

- 1 cup macaroni

- 2 cups shredded cheddar cheese

- Olive oil

- Ritz crackers, crumbled

Method

• Cook macaroni according to package instructions. Drain and set aside.

• Preheat oven to 350 degrees.

• In a frying pan, add olive oil and onions. Fry until onions become translucent.

• Add soup and roughly half of the cheese and mix well. Add in the milk, stirring continuously. Cook on medium heat.

• Add cooked chicken and macaroni and mix well. Add salt and pepper.

• Transfer the chicken and macaroni to a casserole dish lined with Ritz cracker crumbs.

• Bake for 15 minutes until heated through.

• Top with remaining cheese and bake for 5 more minutes.

18.   Bistro Sandwich

(Prep time: 10 minutes. Calories: 301)

Ingredients

- ¾ tbsp thin sliced sun-dried tomatoes

- 1 tbsp red wine vinegar

- Red pepper flakes to taste

- 1 ½ tbsp Neufchatel cheese

- 2 tbsp crumbled feta cheese

- 3 to 5 Greek olives, pitted and chopped

- 3 cloves garlic, crushed

- ½ tsp dried basil

- ¼ tsp sweet red pepper

- 2-4 slices of sourdough or whole grain bread

- ¾ cup chopped spinach

Method

- To make the tomato cheese spread, combine the sun dried tomatoes, vinegar and red pepper flakes. Heat gently over low heat for 3 minutes. In another bowl, beat the two cheeses together and add the tomato vinegar mixture, olives, garlic and dried basil. Use the spread immediately or refrigerate it for up to 2 days.

• To assemble the sandwich, apply the spread over the bread. Add the spinach leaves and sprinkle sweet red pepper. Cut the bread diagonally. Serve.

19.   Mushroom Kale Polenta

(Prep time: 25 minutes. Calories: 305)

Ingredients

- ⅔ cup polenta

- 250g kale

- 500g button mushrooms

- 2 tbsp tamari sauce

- 2 tbsp fresh thyme, chopped

- Juice from ½ lemon

- Olive oil

Method

- Preheat oven to 375 degrees.

- In a saucepan, boil 3 cups of water and add polenta, stirring continuously. Keep stirring until polenta thickens. Place lid on the pan and simmer for 2 minutes on medium heat. Keep stirring from time to time. Cook for 3 more minutes, then turn off heat. Keep the pan covered so the polenta continues to cook.

- Remove the kale stems. Place the leaves in a baking tray with some olive oil, salt and pepper. Bake the leaves for 15 minutes.

- In a frying pan, heat olive oil and fry the mushrooms with tamari sauce and thyme leaves. Sauté for 5-7 minutes.

- Once everything is cooked, add the lemon juice to the polenta.

• To serve, pour the polenta into a deep dish. Add the mushrooms and kale leaves on top.

20.   Tuna Hummus Wrap

(Prep time: 20 minutes. Calories: 280)

Ingredients

- 6 oz can of tuna

- 1 small cucumber, peeled and sliced

- 1 small tomato, sliced

- 2 tbsp olive oil

- 1 tbsp fresh dill

- ¼ tsp pepper

- ⅓ cup hummus

- 8 inch tortilla wraps made of whole wheat

- 4 cups coarsely chopped lettuce

Method:

- Mix together tuna, cucumber, tomato, oil, dill and pepper.

- Spread hummus over each tortilla.

- Divide the tuna filling evenly between the wraps.

- Secure the wraps by folding them. Serve immediately.

Chapter 6: Mediterranean Snack Recipes

These snacks are quick, healthy and delicious. They're the perfect thing to tide you over between meals.

1.   Hummus

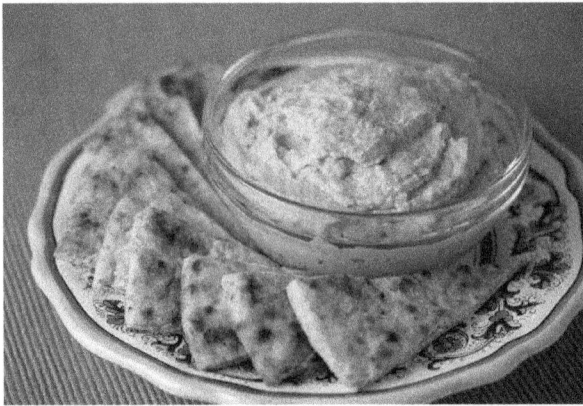

(Prep time: 5 minutes. Calories: 166)

Ingredients

- 1 ½ cup cooked chickpeas
- ½ cup oil
- 1-2 tsp garlic, finely chopped
- ¼ cup lemon juice (optional)
- A pinch of salt

Method

- Chop the chickpeas to remove the outer shell. Don't worry if you do not get all the shells. This gives a nice texture to the hummus.

• Mash the chickpeas with a masher. Add salt, lemon and garlic. Drizzle oil and mix well. Store in refrigerator.

• Serve with pita bread, carrots, celery, rice crackers, etc.

2.   Fruit and Nut Snack Mix

(Prep time: 25 minutes. Calories: 384)

Ingredients

- 1 tbsp butter

- ¼ cup honey

- 1 tsp almond extract

- 1 tsp ground cinnamon

- 2 cups old-fashioned oats

- ½ cup each of almonds, dried banana chips, tropical fruit mix, and raisins

Method

- Preheat oven to 350 degrees.

- In a saucepan, melt butter. Add honey, almond extract and cinnamon. Mix well. Add oats and stir.

- Prepare a baking pan by lining it with parchment paper.

- Transfer the sticky oat mixture to the baking pan and spread it evenly. It should be no more than about 1 inch thick.

- Bake for 10 minutes. Stir in almonds and bake for 5 minutes. Remove from oven. Add the bananas, fruits and raisins. Cool completely before serving.

3.   Grape Smoothie

(Prep time: 5 minutes. Calories: 187)

Ingredients

- 1 cup seedless grapes

- ½ cup each frozen cherries, frozen strawberries, oranges and banana slices

Method

- Blend all ingredients in a blender until smooth. Serve chilled.

4.   Grilled Fruit

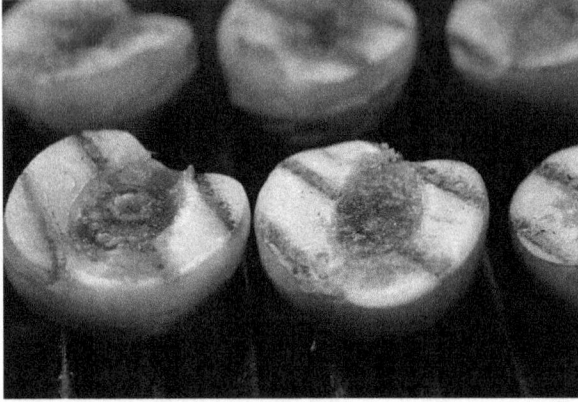

(Prep time: 10 minutes. Calories: 19)

Ingredients

- 4 peaches, plums or nectarines cut in halves

Method

- Grill the fruit in the cooler end of the grill for up to 8 minutes. Turn after 4 minutes. Serve hot.

5.   Tzatziki Dip (Cucumber and Yogurt Dip)

(Prep time: 5 minutes. Calories: 35)

Ingredients

- 1 cup of plain Greek yogurt, low fat

- 2 Lebanese cucumbers, grated and drained

- 2 cloves garlic, minced

- 1 tbsp olive oil

- Salt and pepper

Method

- Mix olive oil and garlic in a bowl.

- Add all the remaining ingredients.

- Serve with asparagus, broccoli, carrots and other vegetables.

Conclusion

The Mediterranean diet is a revolutionary approach to healthy eating. With the guidelines in this book, you can eat like the Greeks and Italians have done since ancient times. By following the Mediterranean diet, not only will you lose weight but you could also look younger and live longer. This plant-based diet with plentiful fruits, vegetables, and whole grains is the path to better heart health and reduced risk of diabetes, hypertension, and other lifestyle diseases. The recipes in this eBook are easy to follow and wonderful to eat. Fruits, veggies, heart-healthy fats, a glass of red wine, and meals enjoyed with friends and family — that is the key to a long, happy life. Enjoy!

I am extremely grateful that you have decided to purchase my book and start improving your health. You even finished the book, well done!

As a thank you I want to send you ANOTHER 20 Mediterranean Diet recipes for you to enjoy absolutely FREE! Simply click the link below to get 20+ more Mediterranean Diet recipes for FREE!

https://mediterraneandietforbeginners.com/freegift

If you found this book to be informative and enjoyed the recipes, I would really appreciate you leaving a review! This will help other buyers sort through the nonsense books out there (and believe me, there are a TON of them) and help guide them to the helpful ones so please take the time to help your fellow readers out! The link to leave your review is here: Leave a Review

Check out my Facebook group, too! It's a fantastic community of people interested in the Mediterranean Diet. Lots of great information, delicious recipes, and great people! https://www.facebook.com/groups/1023957707694936/

[1] http://onlinelibrary.wiley.com/doi/10.1002/ana.20854/full
[1] http://www.drhirani.com/Assets/lyonfinalreport.pdf
[1] http://www.bmj.com/content/337/bmj.a1344.short
[2] http://health.usnews.com/best-diet/mediterranean-diet
[3] https://www.hsph.harvard.edu/obesity-prevention-source/obesity-causes/diet-and-weight/
[4] http://www.medicaldaily.com/heart-health-plan-follows-cardiologist-approved-mediterranean-diet-how-live-and-eat-321902
[5] http://www.webmd.com/vitamins-and-supplements/news/20140512/resveratrol-in-red-wine-may-not-be-such-a-health-booster-after-all
[6] Based on the Lyon Diet Heart study taken from The Everything Mediterranean Diet Book: All you need to lose weight and stay ...By Connie Diekman, Sam Sotiropoulos
[7] http://www.dssimon.com/MM/ACP-mediteranian-diet/Mediterranean Diet with No Fat Restrictions.pdf
[8] http://www.nejm.org/doi/full/10.1056/NEJMoa1200303
[9] http://archinte.jamanetwork.com/article.aspx?articleid=773456
[10] https://www.ncbi.nlm.nih.gov/pmc/articles/PMC3222874/
[11] https://integrativeoncology-essentials.com/2014/02/mediterranean-diet-can-cut-risk-cancer/
[12] http://www.cancerresearchuk.org/about-cancer/cancers-in-general/cancer-questions/can-turmeric-prevent-bowel-cancer

www.ingramcontent.com/pod-product-compliance
Lightning Source LLC
Chambersburg PA
CBHW031903200326
41597CB00012B/525